MEDITATION FOR MEN

***

A Great Way to Relieve Stress and Clear Your Mind

By: Eric Goodfellow

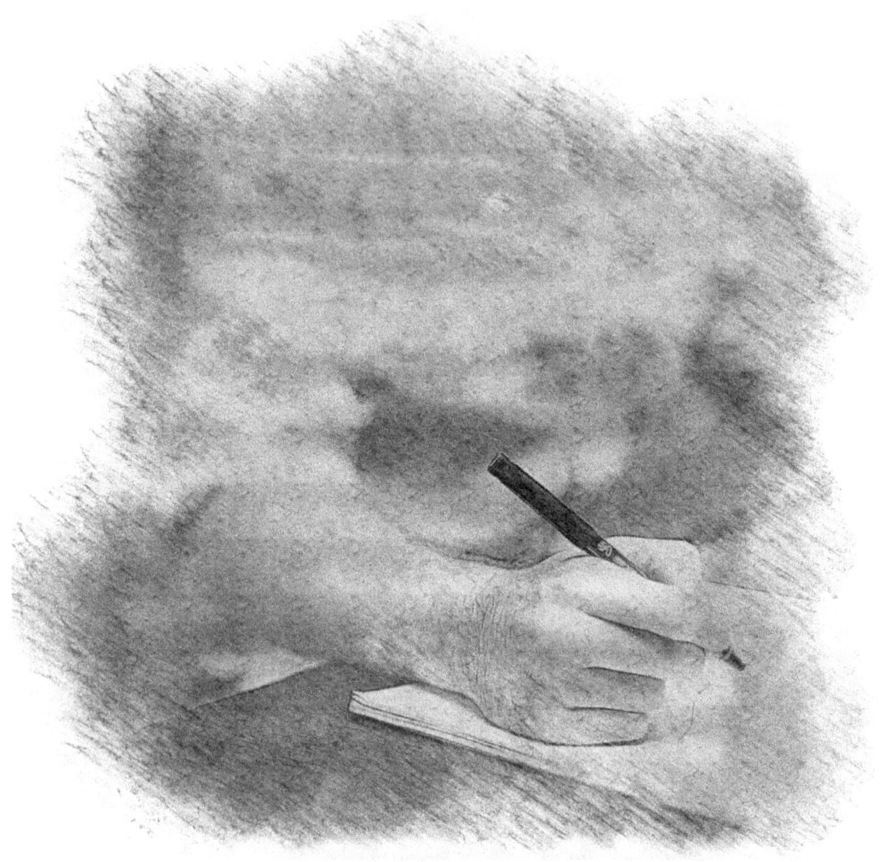

Table of Contents

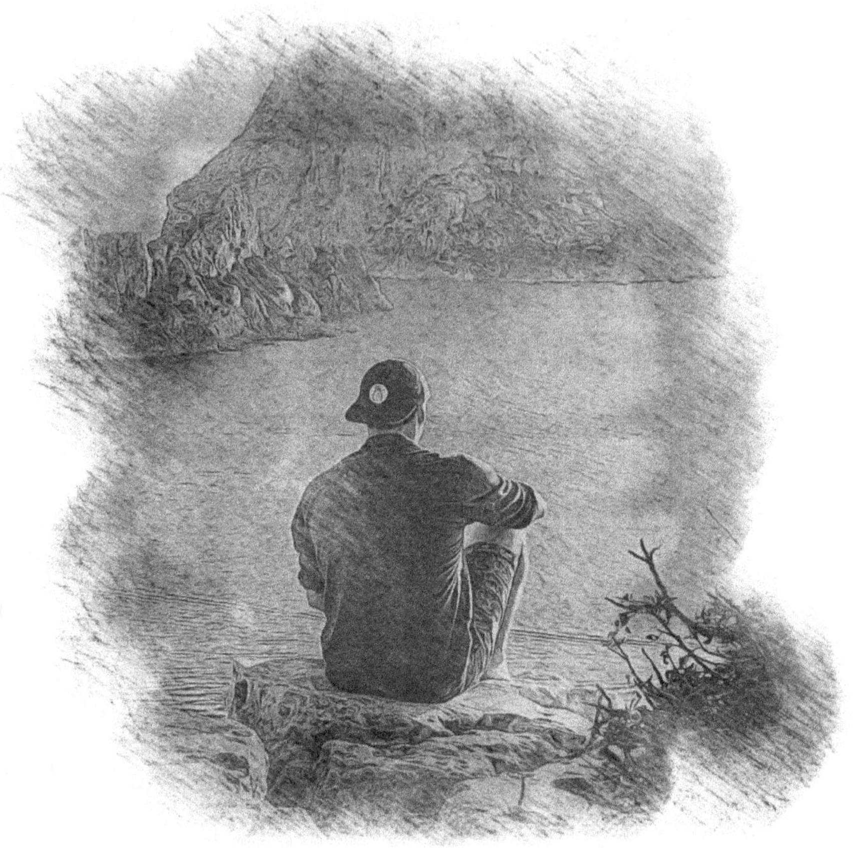

Introduction

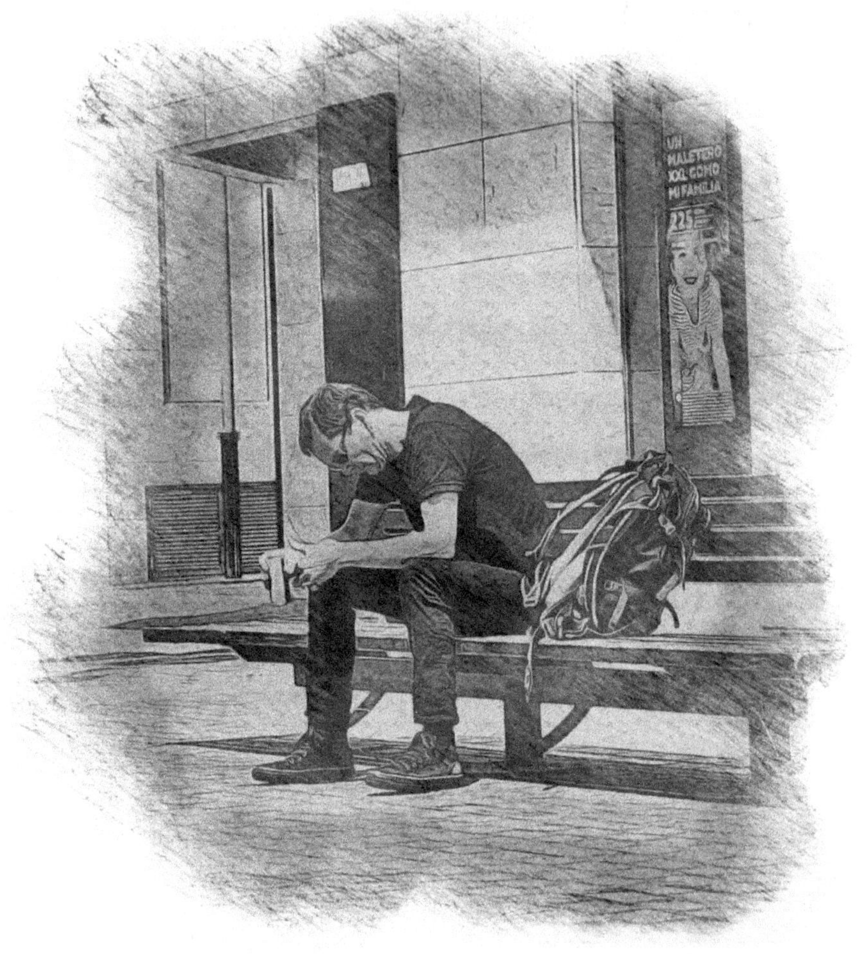

As a man, you are expected to go out and earn money to pay for the lifestyle that you and your loved ones want. The responsibilities are not that different to those that your parents and their parents had but what is different is that today's expectations are more. You find yourself pulled in all directions to keep up with others. You may even find that the materialistic lifestyle that you have been living has caught up with you and you have lost sight of what the original dream was. There are many men today who are looking for a different approach to life, one that gives them back a sense of clarity and the most popular way is by incorporating meditation into your life.

Perhaps it is good to have a little bit of background about what meditation is all about and this book provides it without making it technical. It also shows you how to meditate and gives you clear details of how this can help you in your life. As you may be new to this practice, you need to understand that meditation isn't something that you do on the odd occasion but is something you need to incorporate into your everyday life. I will tell you how to do that because even if you are a man and have a career, it's possible to do it.

Who benefits from meditation?

The truth is that you do and everyone in your entourage does as well. It makes you more patient. It helps you to control your reactions to stress and cuts down a lot of your worry because you start to see life from a different perspective. In fact, as you go through the exercises in this book, you will learn how to meditate, how to use breathing exercises to help you to manage your life better and how to look at life in a totally new way. Are you ready for this adventure? All you need is the will to learn and the patience to find out what life is all about. Meditation opens your eyes. You no longer question your existence because you find the answers easily. This small space of time within each day devoted to meditation helps you to be calm, to be happy and to be able to cope with the stresses of the 21st century in a way that has been used for centuries. Even though the western world did not embrace meditation in early times, people are now finding out for themselves that meditation works. It hones you in on what's important and shuts out the noise of the world for a moment so that you see your life purpose much more clearly.

Meditation can be learned in a class situation together with yoga or can be performed at home on your own, though if you find that you have difficulty at any stage, remember that yoga teachers are trained to help you with your meditation and will be happy to give you further instruction should you need that support. You will also come into contact with like-minded people at a yoga class. Similarly, there are retreat facilities worldwide that help you with the process of learning to let meditation become a part of your life.

Chapter One: Learning to Relax

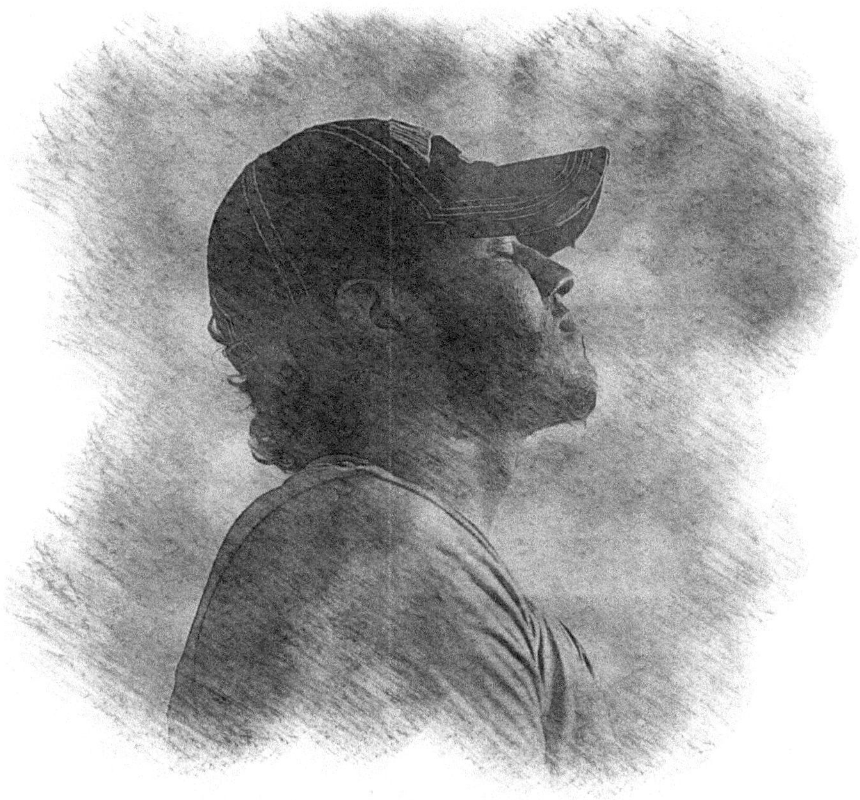

I always begin teaching students to relax because at this time, you probably don't realize how much your breathing affects the life that you live. If you are someone who is stressed easily, then the chances are that you also breathe in too much oxygen, which makes you panic when faced with difficult situations. In the world today, we don't relax. We go from one crisis to the next and simply amble through life hoping for the best. In this body scan exercise, you will learn to switch off the world outside and manage to feel your inner energy increase. Initially, while you are learning to relax, you will find that when you get up and start to live your life after relaxing, you will feel refreshed and happier about your life. Relaxation involves breathing in a way that you are not accustomed to and it's important that you learn this for meditation, since meditation involves being able to concentrate on your breathing and shutting everything else out. Thus, this exercise will help you to move forward with your meditation experience.

You do need to find a time when you won't be disturbed to perform this exercise and since it involves relaxing, I think that the early evening is a good time to perform the exercise. If this means shutting people out of your bedroom, then so be it. Just let family members know that you need a little time to yourself and explain that this is part of your meditation learning process. They will probably be happy to experience a calmer you, so are not likely to object. You have been thinking about work all day and are probably naturally tired, so it's a good time to relax. However, you probably usually spend your evenings with busier things. Today, you need about twenty minutes to yourself and if you want to, you can even involve your partner in the process too.

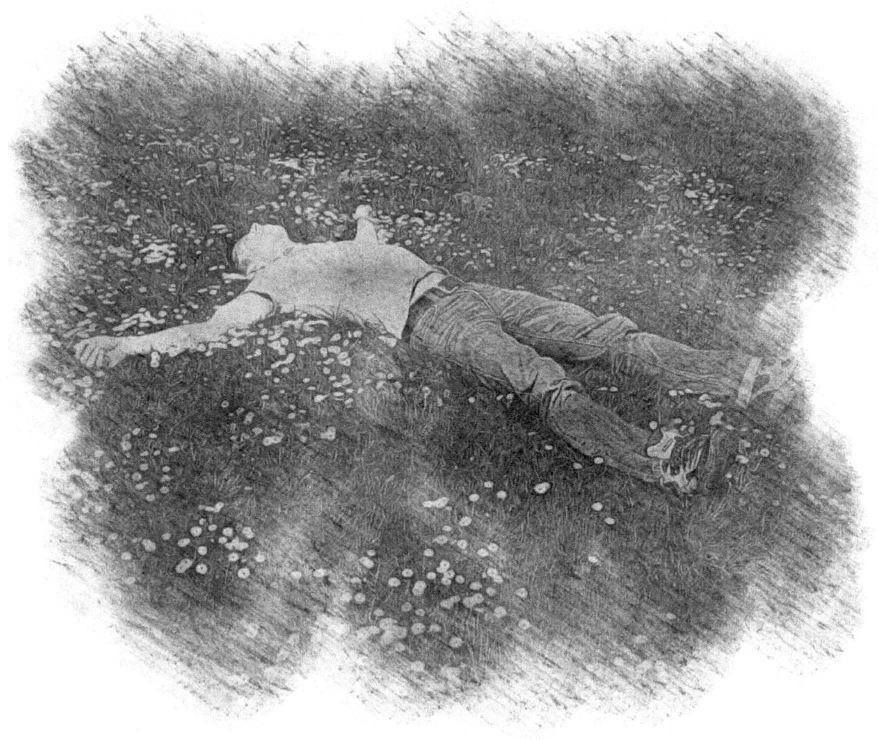

The idea of the body scan is to teach you how to relax. Just like with meditation, you must be dressed in clothing that is not restrictive in any way. Lie down on the bed and use only one pillow. This places your head in the best position so that you can breathe deeply and your airways are optimally placed for the best results. Now, close your eyes because this stops you from being distracted during the process. Breathe in through the nostrils and feel your upper abdomen swell and you breathe in to the count of 8. Now, breathe out to the count of ten.

Keep repeating this until you have a nice rhythm going and then we will start to do the body scan.

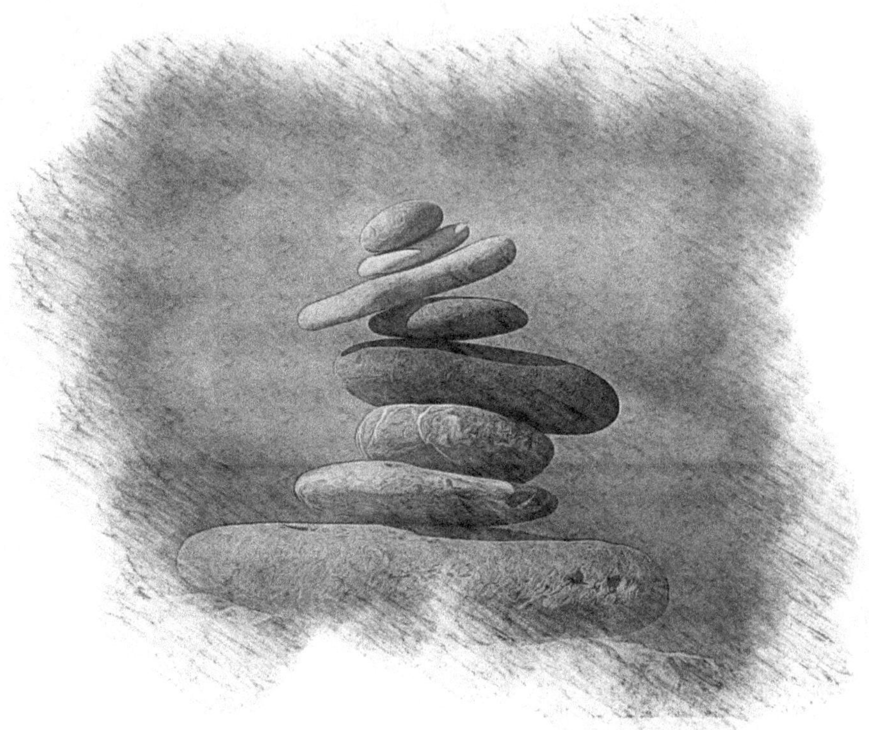

What you do during the body scan is start with your feet. Concentrate fully on your feet while continuing to breathe in the manner I have shown you. Tense your feet and then relax them. Feel them tense up and then feel them relax totally, so that they feel heavy. Move up to your ankles and do the same thing, remembering to tense the area up so that you feel it and then relax it so that it feels heavy – at the same time breathing in the same way as you started.

You work through each area of the body including the following:

Calves, knees, thighs, hips, stomach, chest, shoulders, fingers, hands, wrists, elbows, neck, face, head.

By the time that you have worked your way up the body, you should be totally relaxed and should still be breathing in the same way as you started. Your blood pressure will go down and certainly your heart rate will have decreased. Therefore, don't assume that you can just get up and get on with your day. You need to let your body get back to normal before you do this. The same thing happens when you meditate and the same transition will be required to get back on your feet and get on with your day. Take it slowly. You can use these few moments to reflect on your relaxation session and feel wonderfully refreshed by it.

What you have learned is to concentrate your thoughts on given things and that's where meditation starts. During meditation, you won't be concentrating on a separate area of the body, but you will be concentrating on the breath. That's why I have introduced you to this method of breathing. When you think about it, it's a known fact that when human beings breathe, they don't use the full capacity of the lungs but only a very small amount of that capacity. When you breathe more deeply, you allow your sympathetic nervous system to work in a more efficient way, meaning that the controls of being hot or cold are more efficient and the spread of oxygen to all of your muscles is a natural follow on.

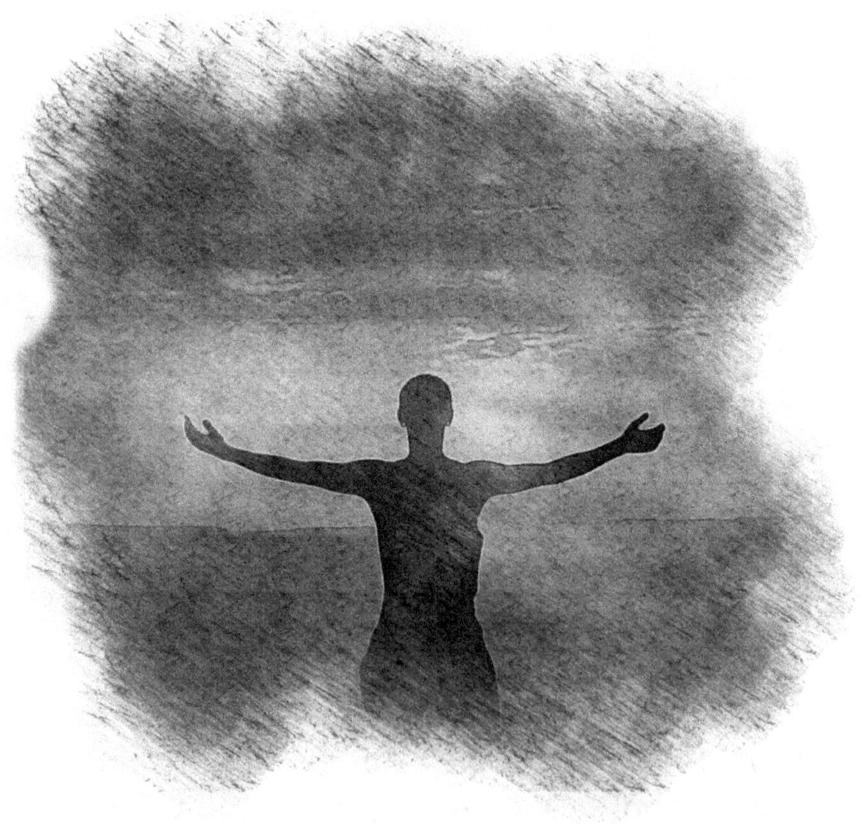

How often you do this exercise is up to you, although it's a great exercise to perform after you have had a warm shower and are relaxed naturally.

This gives you the edge and helps you to drift off while you scan the body and leads to the ability to meditate because meditation is just one step further than the relaxation exercise. During meditation, you won't be honing in on body parts, but will be concentrating on your breath or nothing at all. When you consider the amount of information the human mind is exposed to during a lifetime, you will also understand that meditation allows you to step away from this bombardment and allow the subconscious mind to be able to solve all of your problems without interference from outside influences.

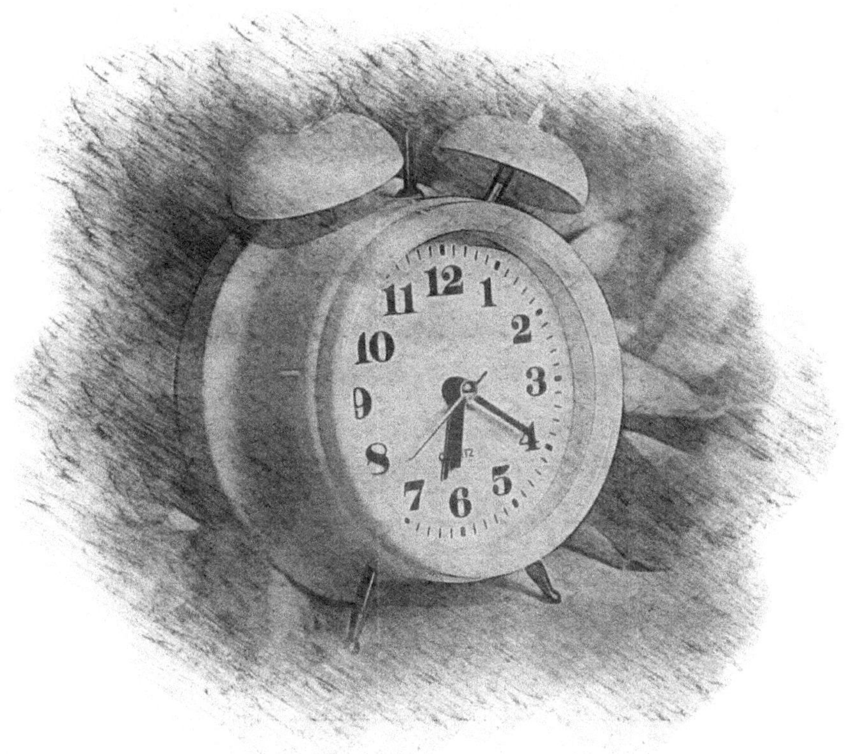

As well as learning to meditate, you also need to appreciate that your body needs the three elements of work, rest and play in equal proportions. Sleeping well at night is vital because this allows your body and mind to regenerate and heal from all the work and toil that you have exposed it to. Eating the right kinds of foods also helps you to feel better about your life and you will find that meditation will veer you toward looking after yourself in a better way than you may have done up until now. Learn to listen to your body because the messages it is sending to you are purposeful and express the needs of the body. When you learn to listen to them, you improve your life no end. You can use the relaxation technique shown above at any time that you feel you need to switch off from the busy world and it will help to set your mind at peace and rest your body in the way that it needs. However, this does not replace the need for 8 hours sleep per night.

Chapter Two: Preparing your Home for Meditation

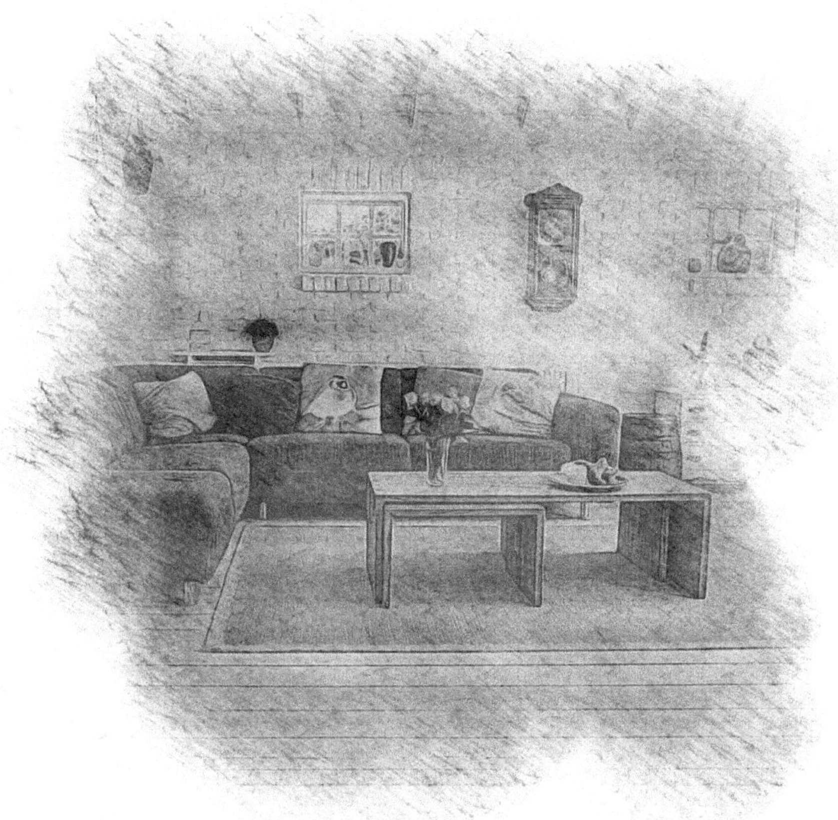

Meditation needs space. If you create a space specifically for meditation, it is logical that you will want to use that space on a regular basis. Since you need to meditate for about 20 minutes a day at first, this commitment to creating a space is quite important and logical. The kind of things that you will need are as follows:

- Comfortable clothing that does not restrict you
- A comfortable chair
- Or a yoga mat and a stool for meditation

Other things that you add to this space are completely up to you. However, many find that having inspirational items in this area helps them to remember why they are meditating in the first place. For example, you may want to have a statue of Buddha or something equally inspirational. You may not know it, but Buddha was the founder of the philosophy that we now know as Buddhism and he reached enlightenment – which is a direct result of perfect meditation. What he wanted to know about was what could be done to stop mankind from suffering and it was during this enlightenment that he found the answers. Your questions or your problems in life may be different to his, but you are equally able to use meditation to find clarity. You are allowing your mind silence and that's something that the 21st century does not allow. Thus, when you have a statue of Buddha, it isn't used as something to worship. It is more likely that you find inspiration and that's what the Buddha statues are intended to give you.

If you go into Buddhist temples, you will find that the altars are colored in pastel shades and that there is a great deal of ornament and decoration. Unlike altars in churches, which bear images or symbols that people worship, your altar or inspirational area in your home only has to have things that you believe will help in your meditation practice. You may want to take inspiration from scents and people often use incense to create the atmosphere that helps them to meditate. A vase of your favorite flowers can do the same thing. However, the area that you create for meditation gives you that little bit of commitment to a daily practice and makes it more likely that you will stick to your meditation.

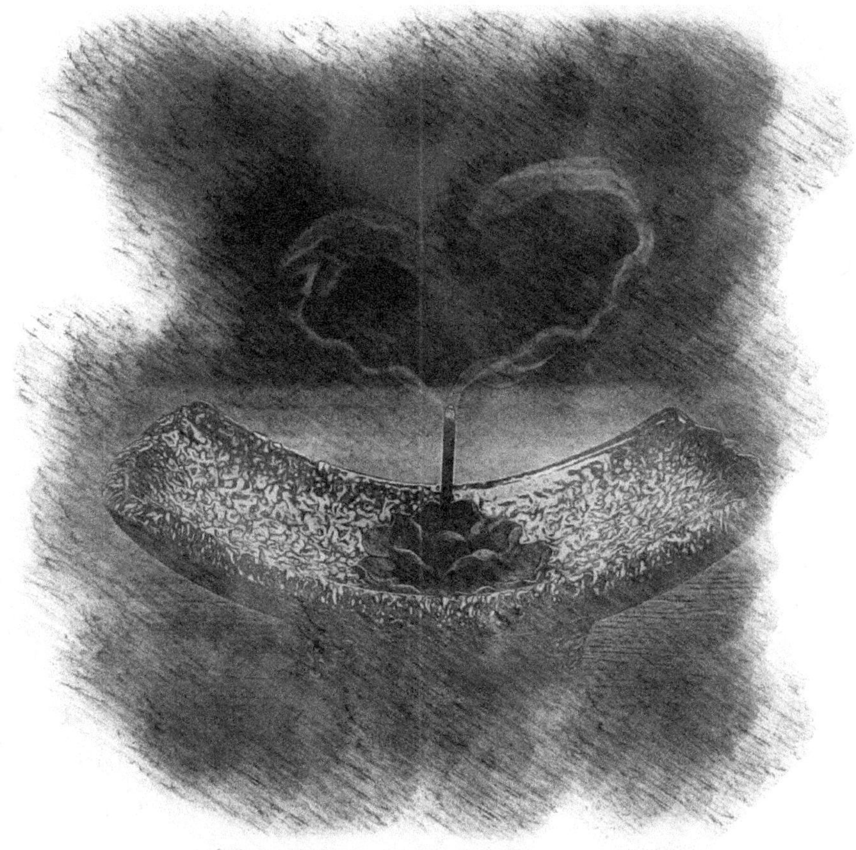

It's creating a space for a specific purpose and men tend to see things in black and white and thus this is a very good way of setting yourself up for your future meditation.

Something that works well in conjunction with meditation for a busy man is to put aside time each week to get close to nature. Perhaps you work in the city and don't take any time out to appreciate your surroundings. If you can make sure that you take your lunch hour during the week and get out into a local park, this helps you to appreciate the here and now. Mindfulness goes alongside meditation and what this means is that you step off the roundabout of busyness and step into the moment in which you are. All of this helps you with your meditation and is preparation for meditation. For example, when you sit on a park bench, you try to put thoughts out of your mind that does not relate to this instant. If you had a row in the office today, you don't dwell on it, but you try to let it go, in favor of using your senses to enjoy the moment that you are in.

One of the most difficult things for men to do is to let go. During meditation, you will need to learn to do this and so this little outing each day to a park or natural environment will help you to be able to do that. Instead of using judgment, you learn to use your senses. It's not a matter of who's to blame for a situation. You should be more concerned about how you feel in this very moment and what your senses are telling you. Your sense of smell, touch, taste, hearing and sight are all there for a purpose, but we forget how to use them. Thus, when something happens that usually has you in a rage, try to let it go. The inner rage is there because you choose to judge something or someone and mindfulness take you from that rage into the moment where you are currently and stops you from using judgment that makes your thoughts dark and negative.

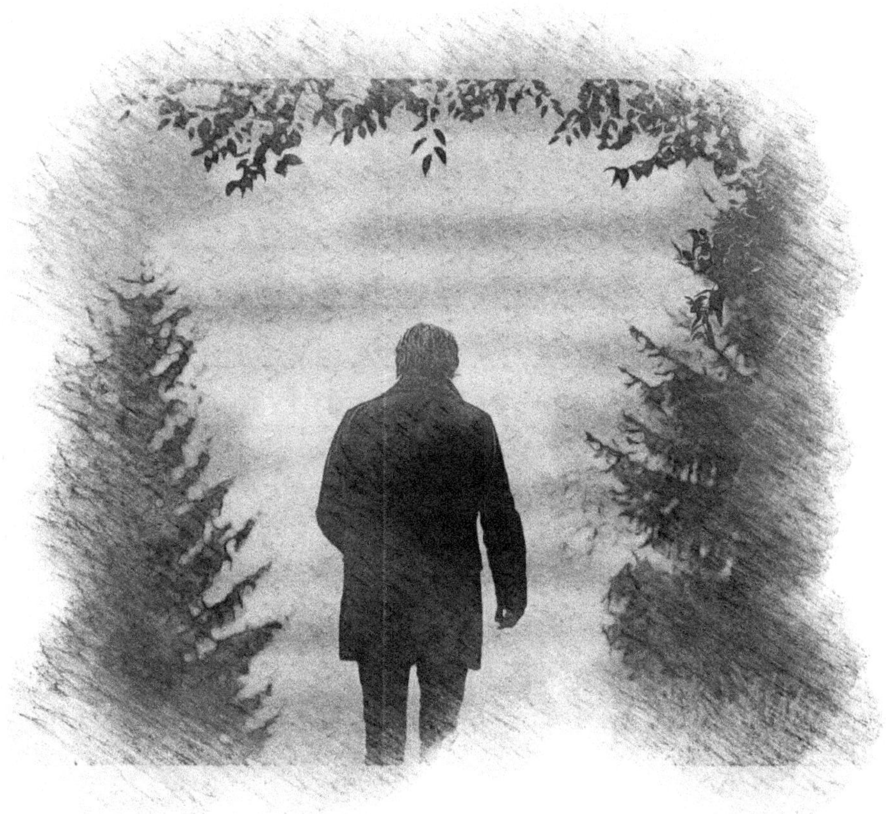

Your thoughts usually veer on the side of negativity. If you practice being in the moment, you let go of all of those concepts and are able to see things from a much clearer viewpoint. It strengthens you and it makes you much more capable of being able to put up with all of the external influences in your life, so that your concentration is better and you are able to find solutions, rather than adding fuel to the fire of life. It also helps to make you more compassionate and you tend to be able to empathize and realize that what people say or do may be fueled by their own problems and that there's not much point in taking in all of that negativity when you don't know the other side of the story. You may think this is going off the subject of meditation, but it works hand in hand with the way that your mind processes thoughts during the course of meditation, so is part and parcel of the experience.

Another preparation for meditation is getting up close to nature. If you have the opportunity to go somewhere where the countryside awes you, this helps you to remember how small you are in the order of things but how vital each small thing is when making up the landscape that you consider inspirational. Imagine a grain of sand. Now imagine a beach without each grain of sand and there would not be a beach. Therefore, each part of the world you live in is to be respected including your mind and body.

Chapter Three: Setting Time Aside to Meditate

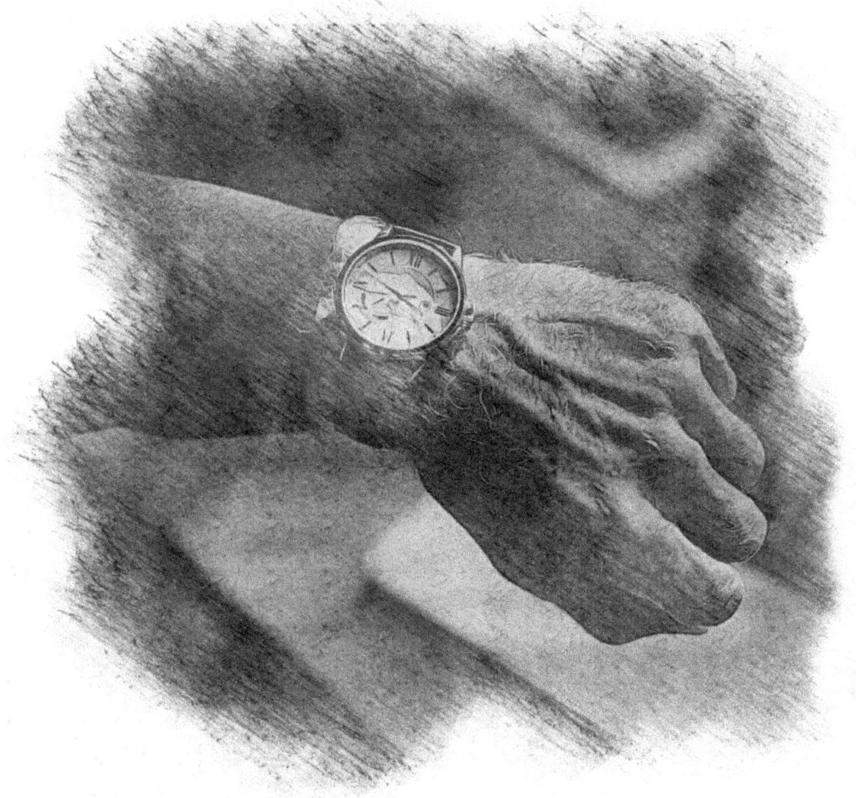

When you decide to start on your meditation journey, you need to set aside time to meditate. The times that are not great for meditation are just after eating because your digestive systems will keep you aware of too much information at a time when you need to let go. Thus, the best times to meditate are either first thing in the morning, before everyone else is up, or early in the evening before your evening meal. Personally, I find that first thing in the morning is best because your mind is not overtaken by thoughts of things that have happened during a stressful day.

It's a good idea to set your alarm clock about half an hour earlier than usual. Get out of bed and do the necessary if you need to go to the toilet and then take up your position for meditation, which is explained below.

Sitting position for meditation

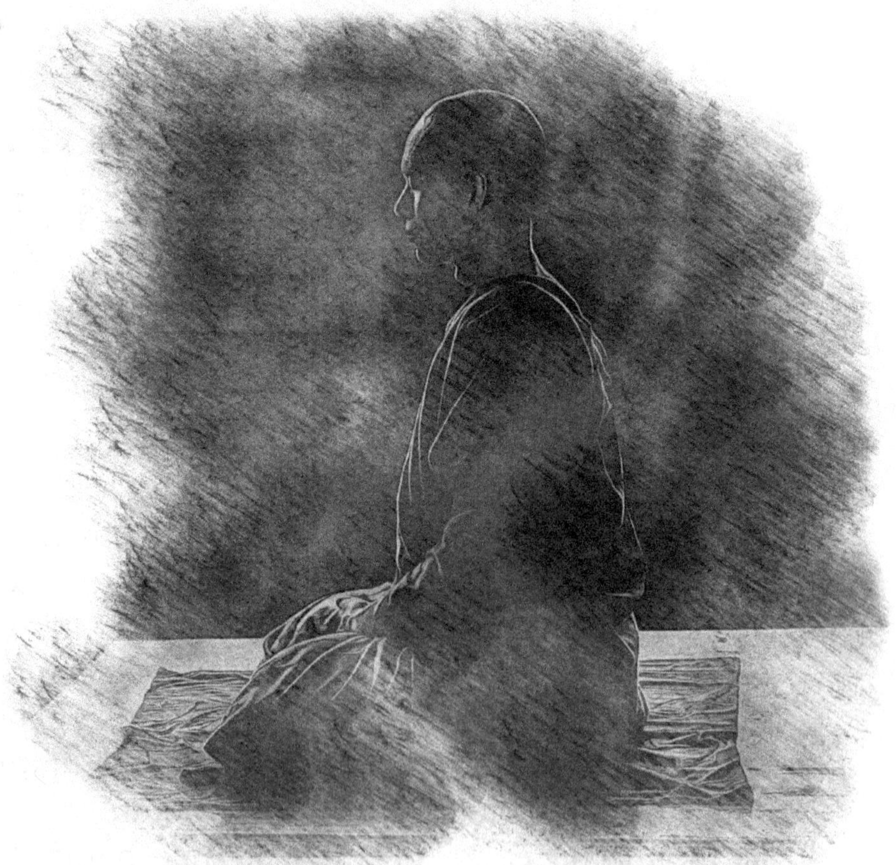

This depends upon how fit you are. If you find it

hard to get down onto a yoga mat, then use a chair, but make sure that the chair is a solid one like a dining chair that encourages your back to be straight. You may not be aware of it, but energy flows through your body all of the time. If there are blockages, then this energy cannot reach all of the places it needs to reach. During meditation, you are asked to sit with your feet flat on the floor (if using a chair). Your back should be straight and your head slightly bowed. Your right hand (if right handed) should support your left hand and the palms should face upward with your thumbs touching each other. There's a very good logical reason for this and it is that you are not encouraged to distract your mind from the meditation process. Your feet on the floor ground you to the earth so that you are unlikely to move. Your hands, similarly, are occupied doing something so are unlikely to be moving during the meditation process.

If you are sitting on your meditation stool on the yoga mat, then your knees should be bent and your ankles crossed. Don't expect to get into a lotus position unless you have been trained to do so during yoga classes. It's too difficult and can be painful. Your hands should be similarly placed as they are when you are using a chair as described above.

The Breathing that leads to meditation

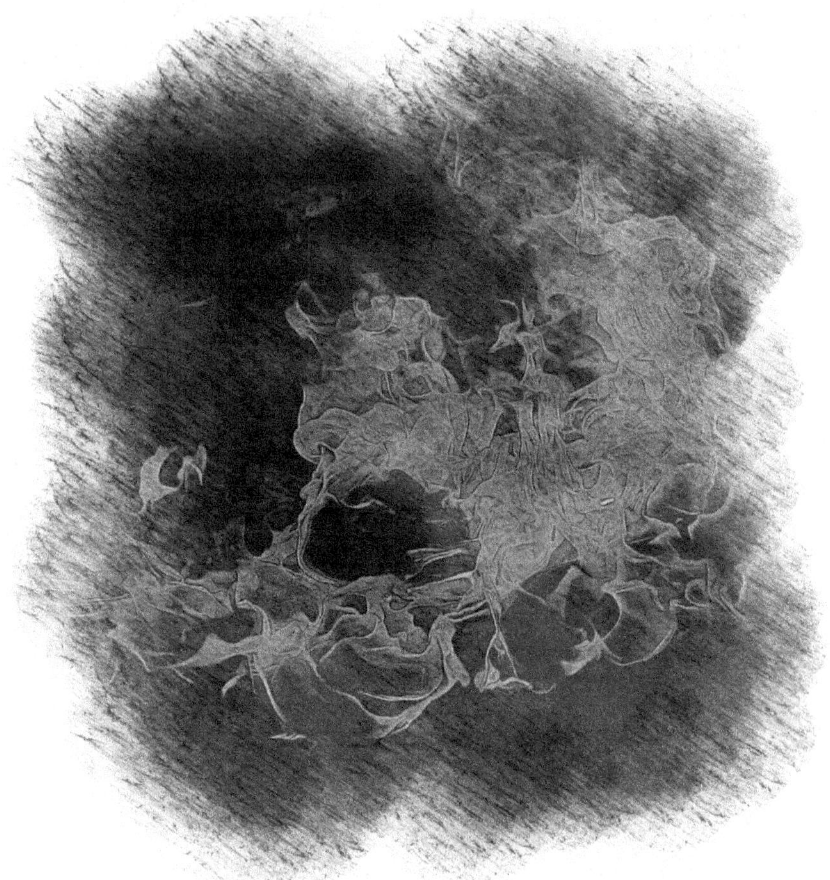

This is quite important. Breathe in through your nostrils to the count of 8. Feel the air going into your body and try to concentrate only on your breathing. If it helps you at all, you can imagine the breath in some tangible way, such as flames going into your body. Feel the air entering your body and feel the upper abdomen rise. Breathe out to the count of 10, feeling your body release that air and letting go of it as you count toward ten.

The above inhale and exhale counts as ONE. The idea is to do this repeatedly until you get to ten when you start over at one again. However, in the early stages of meditation, you will find that the mind gets distracted. Each time it does and you get thoughts come into your mind, you must go back to one again.

Getting rid of thoughts

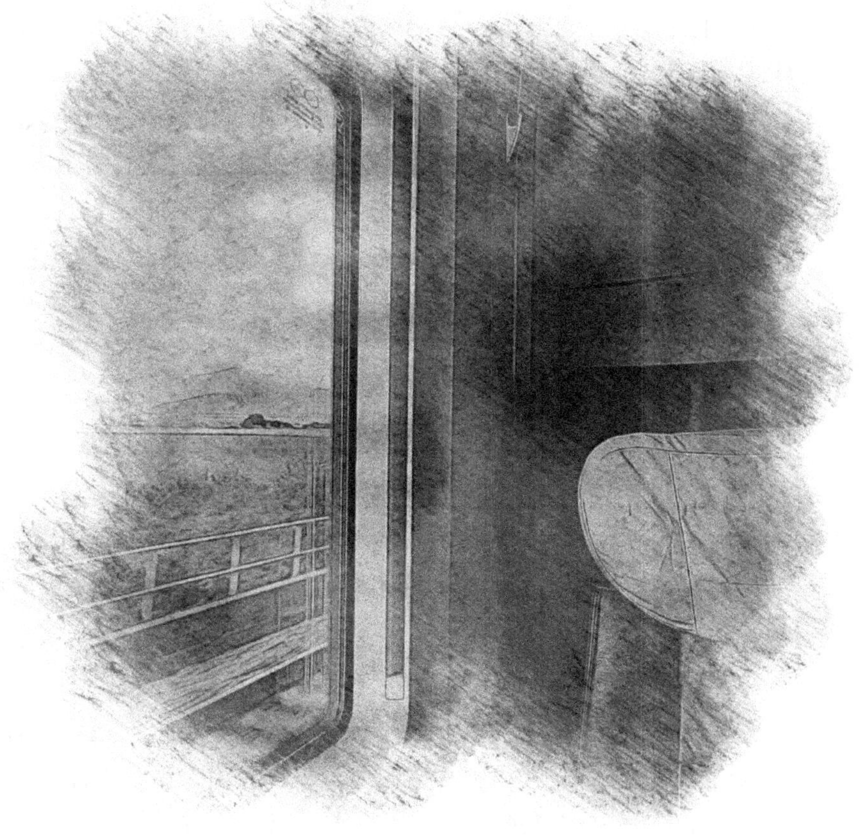

Since you are accustomed to having random thoughts, it's not that easy to let go. Don't expect great things of yourself in the early stages of learning to meditate. Thoughts will come into your mind, but instead of attaching emotions to them, you need to see them as if they are simply detached from you. Imagine them perhaps like images that you see from the window of a train. They come and go and the most important element is that you must attach no judgment to them whatsoever. See them as balloons if you want to and let them drift off into the sky. The idea of lack of judgment is that all of your life, as a man who is trying to do his best for his life and family, you are always surrounded by thoughts and plans. While you are meditating, this is not the case. You are entitled to freedom from these thoughts and conclusions. All that exists during your meditation session is the breath.

Effort

All of your working life or in fact all of your growing up life, you have been encouraged to do your best. Therefore, when thoughts get in the way of meditation, you may consider yourself as a failure. However, there is no failing. There is no real success either. The thing that you need to get your head around is that there's no effort needed. You simply need to BE in that moment while you meditate and in fact, the harder you try, the less likely you are to be able to meditate since meditation is letting go of all of these concepts and simply being within yourself. We don't often get to look inside ourselves because the world insists that we look at what's going on around us. Thus, it's very hard at the beginning to get your head around what meditation is. It is merely a question of BEING.

How does that help you? When you breathe in the manner suggested and you simply BE, you are getting closer to who you are as a human being. You are not trying to be something. You are merely BEING who you are. I can't emphasize this enough. It's a relaxation and almost a trance state where nothing around you matters and you get close to the link between mind and body. People who have been through enlightenment as a result of their meditation describe it as an opening up of their understanding beyond the realms of what we would normally understand. However, enlightenment isn't going to be your aim. Your aim is simply to BE.

Chapter Four: Exercises in Meditation

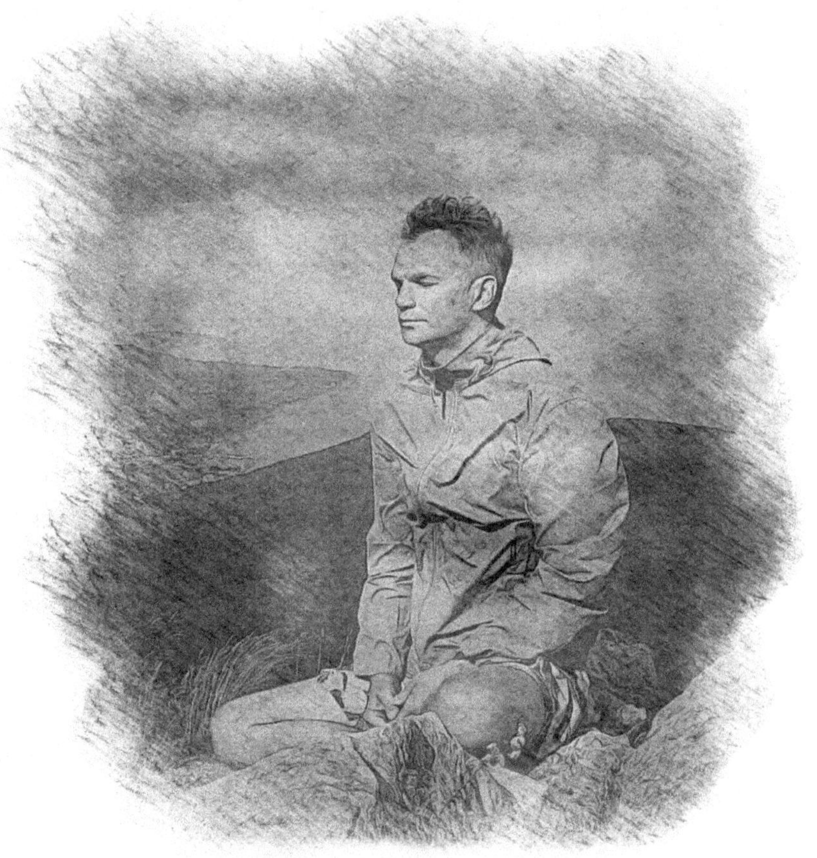

In the last chapter, we showed you what meditation is. It's a physical thing that you do in order to discover what lies beyond the scope of human understanding of self. You begin to see life in a much clearer way. You learn patience and you respect the body that you live in. All of this may sound a little strange to a man who has never meditated before, but when you incorporate this into your life, it lifts your life to such an extent that:

- You can control the way that you respond to life
- You have a better understanding of self
- You are more compassionate toward others
- You find solutions to life's problems
- You are more aware than you ever have been

So how can all of these benefits be brought into your everyday life as a working man? Well, the answer lies in doing exercises to help you to gain clarity. For example, if you have an interview ahead and are worried about it, meditation exercises will help to calm you. Let's face it; if you go for a job interview with nervousness as a key element in your mind, then the interviewers are going to notice that nervousness. However, when your mind is cleared of doubt and you enter an interview room, you come over as being secure in who you are and are much more likely to win over the positive praise of those who will decide your future. Let's look at some exercises you can use during the day to help you to manage yourself and to calm the mind and help you to have better concentration powers.

Exercise One:
Walking Meditation

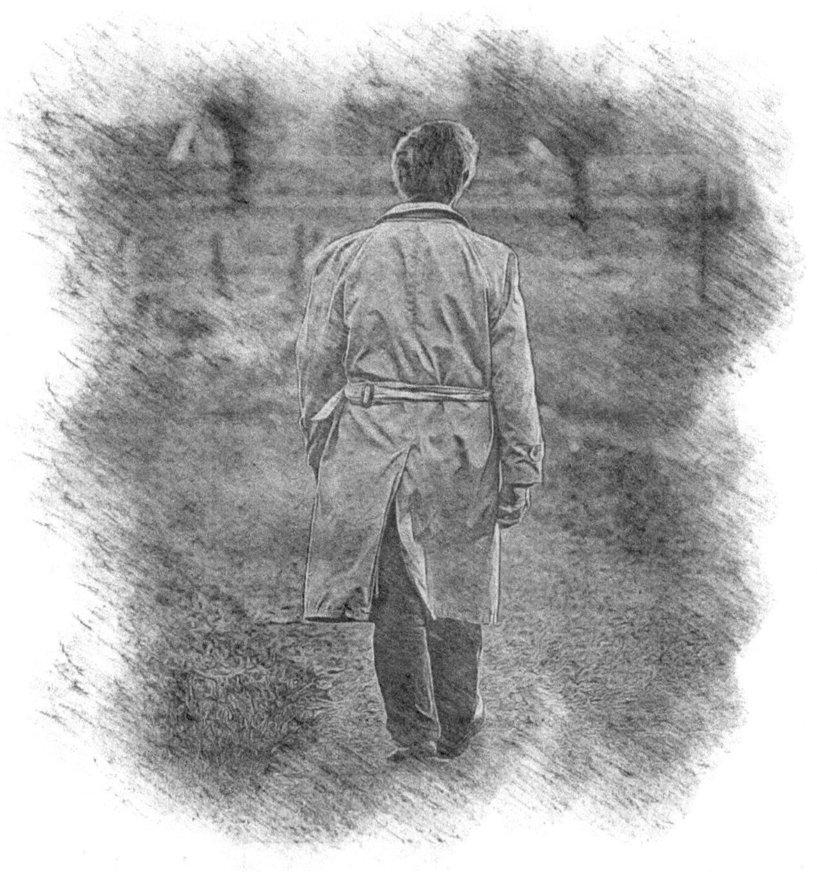

This type of meditation is useful before a meeting. It helps you to prepare your mind for concentrated effort because it doesn't allow the mind to wander off or get filled with negativity. If you have a meeting and are prepared for it, then you can use walking meditation to help you to enter that meeting with a clear mind so that you are able to address the meeting with confidence and clarity.

Go to a place where you can walk up and down or even around in large circles without being bothered too much by your surroundings. You may want to use the car park, a local park or recreation area. In this kind of meditation, your concentration is placed upon the movement of your legs as you walk. You breathe deeply and start to move your leg forward. As the foot touches the ground, you exhale, taking the next breath when you lift your next foot ready to take the next stride. You notice the movement of your feet, the bending of the knee and you concentrate solely on those movements and your breath. Do not be pulled out of that moment. Of course, in this instant, you need to keep your eyes open because otherwise there may be hurdles, but people who do this for several moments before a meeting find that their thoughts are not clouded and that their minds are much clearer. This helps in the meeting because you don't fumble with your words and notes and know exactly where the meeting is heading.

Exercise Two:

Breathing

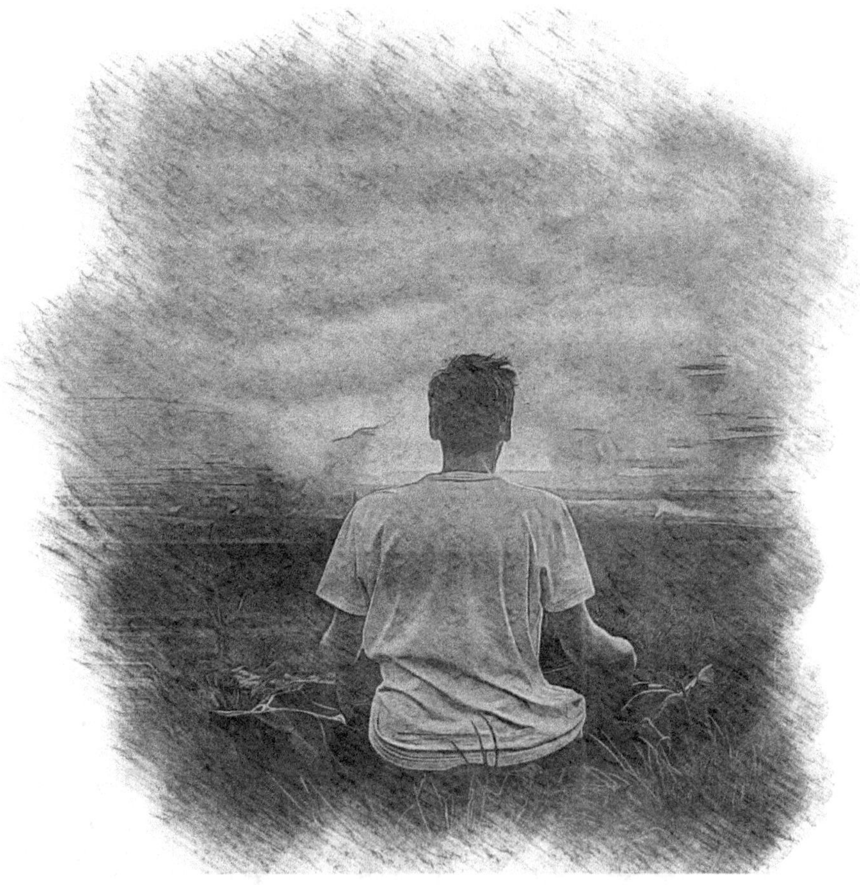

You already know how to breathe for meditation. However, there are other breathing methods that help you to gain clarity when all else fails. Alternate nostril breathing is one of these. If you can find somewhere private and sit down, place your thumb against one nostril and breathe in deeply through the other. You can use the same counting method as you use for meditation if you like but choose what is comfortable for you. Breathe in through the open nostril, hold the air inside you for a moment while you switch over to holding the other nostril closed and allowing the air to be pushed out through the first nostril. So, you are breathing in through one nostril and then breathing out through the other. Then breathe in through the same nostril and breathe out through the other. Do this about a dozen times but all the time that you are doing it, stay focused on just your breathing and don't let thoughts get in the way of what you are doing. This allows your mind to have sufficient oxygen but it also helps to build up your clarity by getting rid of toxins, which may be in your breath, and you really will feel more energetic mentally when you have done the exercise. Practice it at home if you want to see how it works because it helps you considerably and you can do this anywhere as a means of calming yourself down and honing in on those important things you may have to deal with in the next hour or so.

Remember that when you lose your temper, or you feel that your blood pressure is rising, you can use these exercises to bring it back under control. You can also use the relaxation method that I described in Chapter One to help you to regain your composure and to feel calm again. These are useful tools in this day and age when there is so much pressure on men to perform in the workplace and to balance their work and home lives without one impinging on the other. The amount of stress in the world today is phenomenal and by using these exercises, you can make your life much easier and learn through meditation to be more comfortable with who you are. Clearing your mind is important when you consider all of the distractions of life and all of the responsibilities a man has to bear in this day and age. Stepping away from technology and being able to relax and breathe will help you to see things from a better perspective and be happy with the part that you play in the workplace and the home.

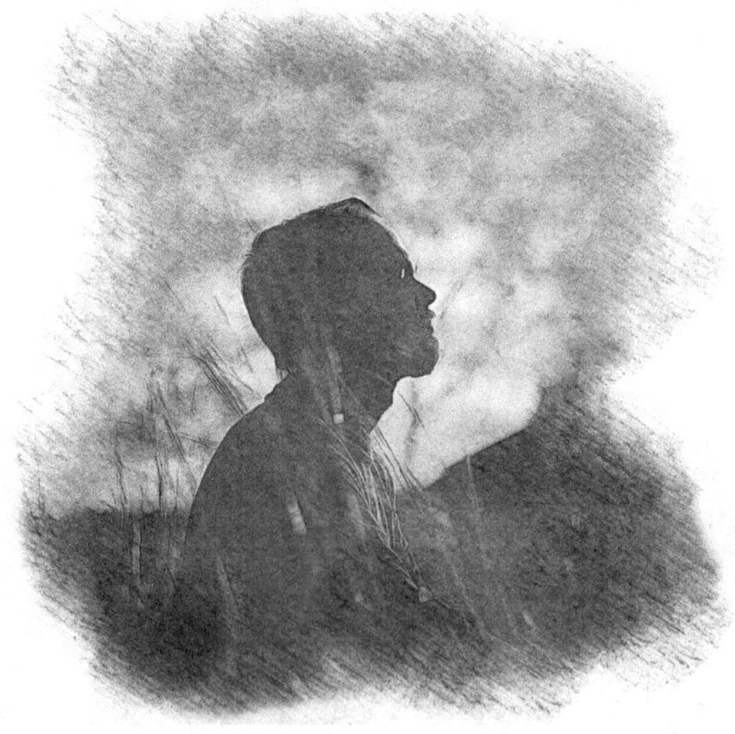

Conclusion

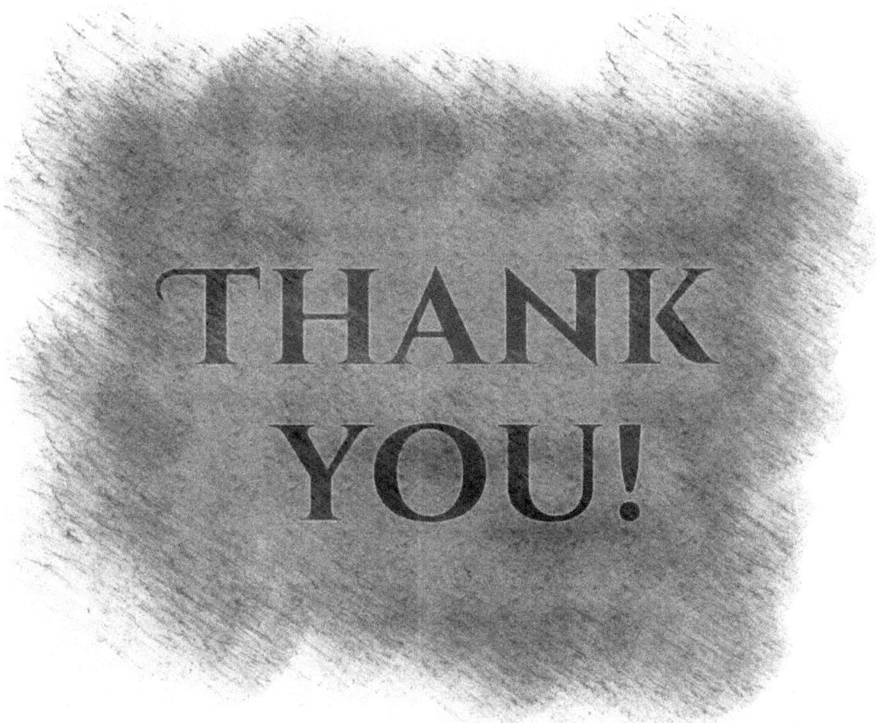

I have taken you through learning to meditate, step by step, because I know that meditation works. It helps you to manage your life. It helps you to see things clearly. It also helps you to collect your thoughts and know which ones are of importance and which ones will hold you back. Remember that negativity helps no one. When the original Buddha, Siddhartha Gautama meditated on why human beings suffer so much, he came up with a menu for life, which is today known as Buddhism. It involved an eight fold path that includes the basic rules to help you to step away from suffering and this included the following elements:

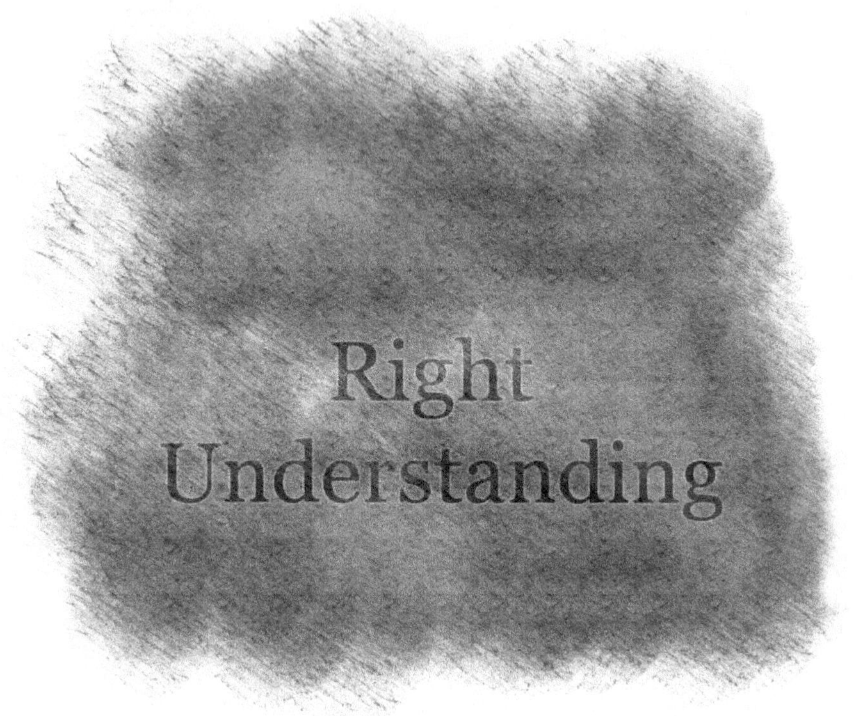

Right Understanding

—

That means not misinterpreting things.

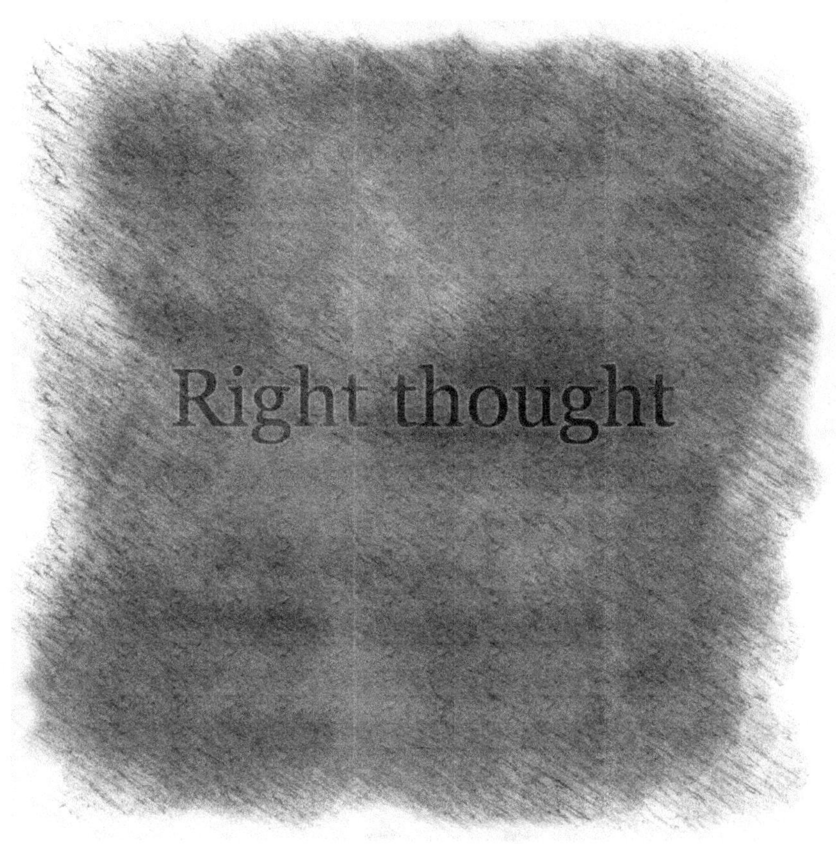

Right thought

—

**That means trying to keep
negative thoughts at bay.**

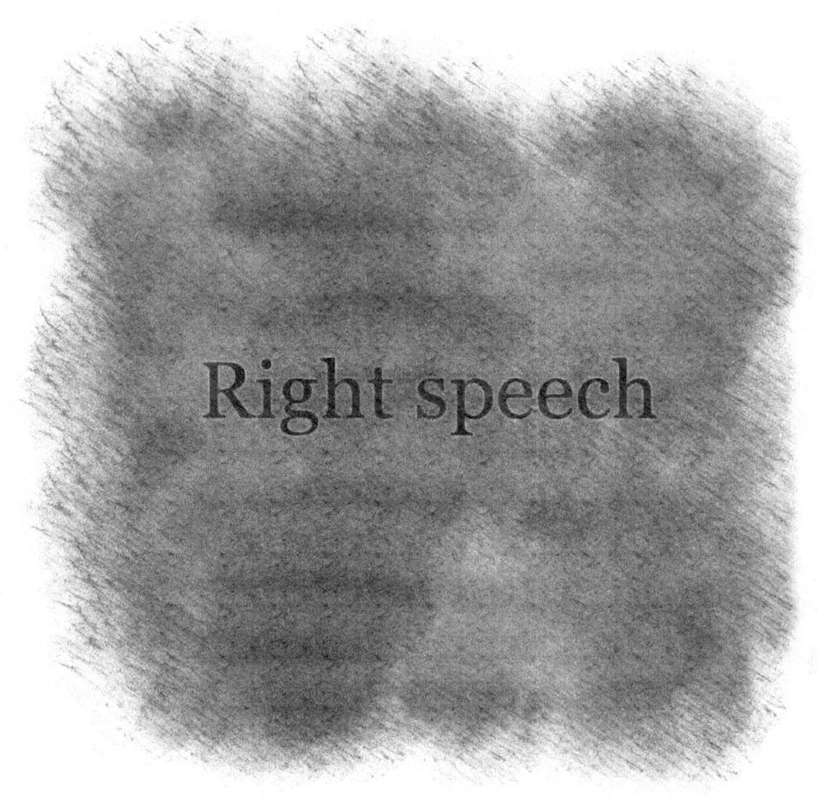

**Right speech
–
That meant saying the right
thing.**

Right Action

—

That meant doing the right thing.

Right Livelihood
—
Meaning that your work should be within your moral belief framework

Right Effort

—

That may seem obvious, though it also means knowing where the effort needs to be exerted.

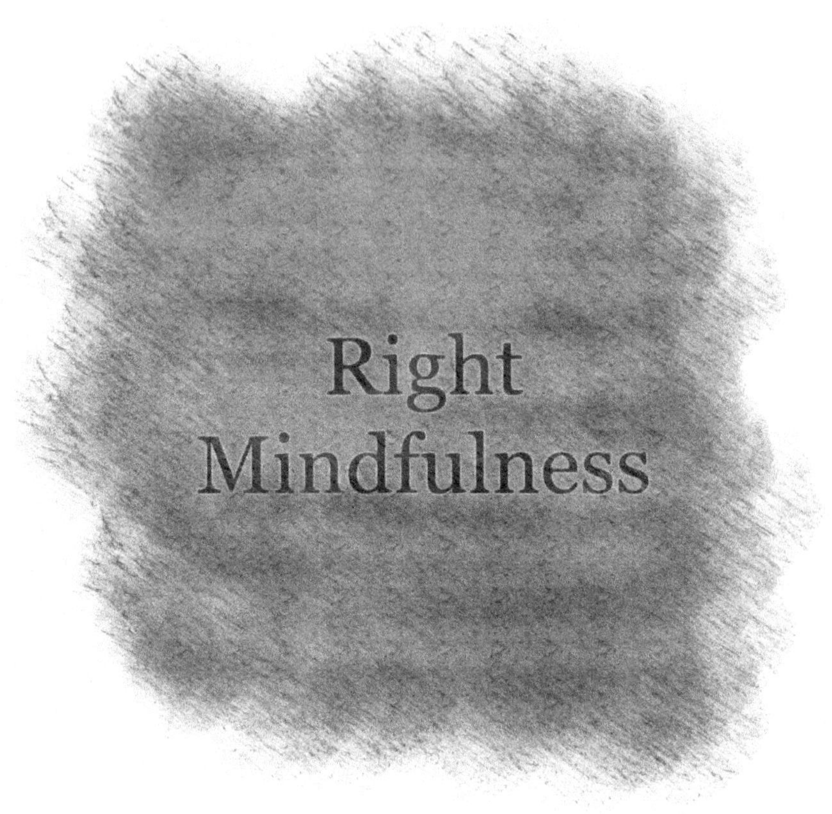

Right Mindfulness

—

**Being aware of who you are
and this moment in time in
your life.**

Right Concentration

Right Concentration

–

That means putting your energies into the right areas of your life.

If you bear these things in mind when you approach your meditation, they help you to live a life, which is devoid of suffering, and thus be able to enjoy your life more. It wasn't his intention to promote any kind of religion at all. The philosophy thus applies to anyone of any religion and when you apply these basic rules to your life – together with practicing meditation – you find that you have clarity and purpose and that you see things in a very different way.

I hope that this book has opened your eyes to possibilities. If it has not, then I suggest you try the exercises that are explained in the book and try to meditate for at least 20 minutes each day. As this becomes a habit, you will find that your life improves and you become mentally stronger than you have ever been. As a man, it's important to have balance in your life and meditation allows this to happen.

My Other Book

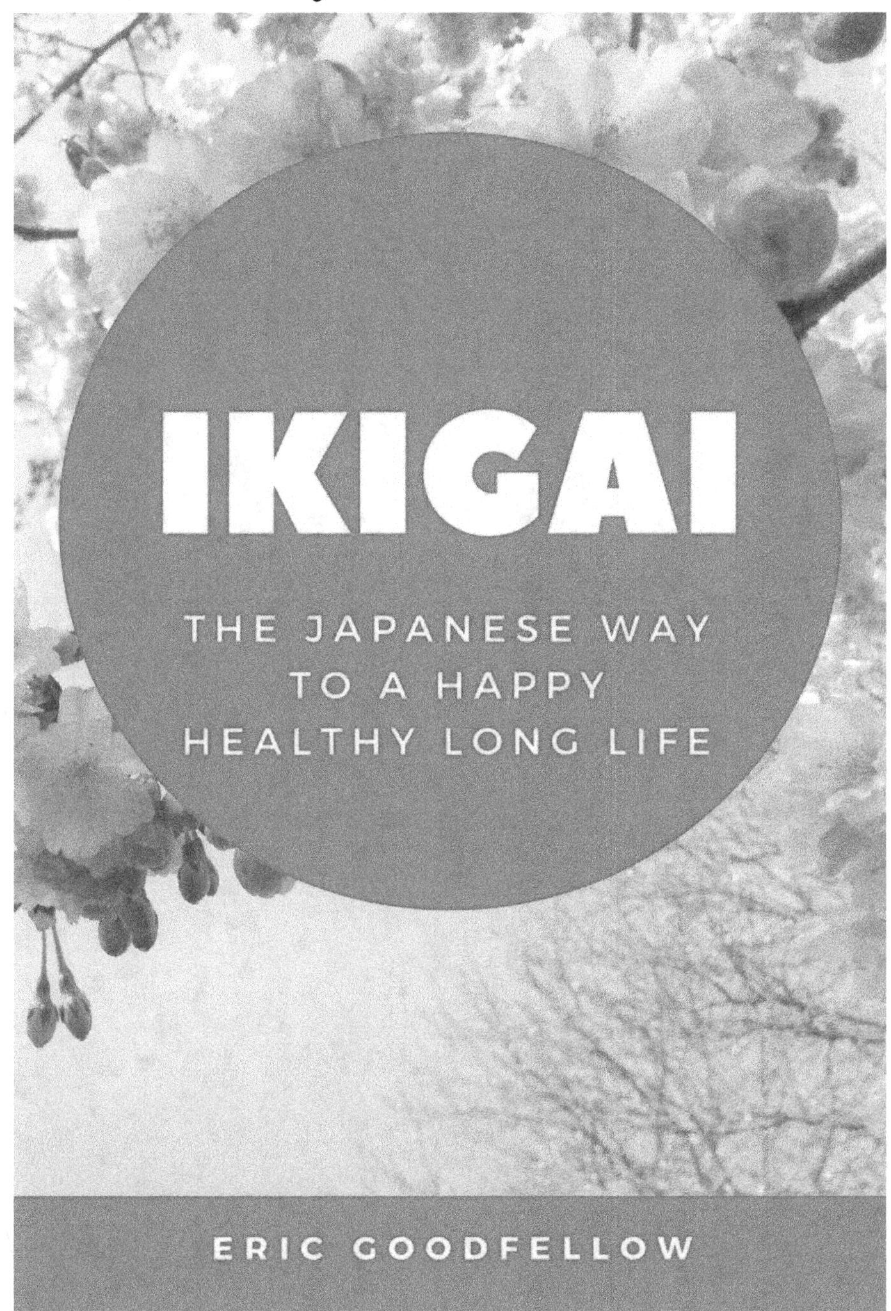